I'VE GOT TO TELL SOMEBODY

A Spiritual Journey Through the Life of a Great Woman of God - A 24 Year Cancer Survivor

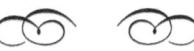

by
Fannie B. Bush

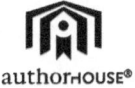

authorHOUSE®

AuthorHouse™
1663 Liberty Drive, Suite 200
Bloomington, IN 47403
www.authorhouse.com
Phone: 1-800-839-8640

First published by AuthorHouse   11/17/2008

ISBN: 978-1-4343-6250-6 (sc)

Printed in the United States of America
Bloomington, Indiana

This book is printed on acid-free paper.

-MY TESTIMONY-

Psalms 118:17–18 "I will not die but live to declare the works of the Lord. God has chastened me sore but he has not given me over to death."

THAT'S WHY I'VE GOT TO TELL SOMEBODY!

Tis so sweet to trust in Jesus, just to take Him at His word, just to rest upon his promise just to know thus said the Lord. Jesus, Jesus! How I trust Him! How I've proved Him o'er and o'er! Jesus, Jesus, precious Jesus! Oh for grace to trust Him more. "THAT'S WHY I'VE GOT TO TELL SOMEBODY."

The spirit of the Lord is upon me. He has anointed me to write my testimony in spirit and in truth. I pray with all of my heart and all that is within me that millions of people will come to know Jesus, my Jehovah Rapha (Our Healer) as I have come to know Him. "THAT'S WHY I'VE GOT TO TELL SOMEBODY."

BOOK DEDICATIONS

To my Great Jehovah-rapha - MY Healer and my Strong Tower

To: My Loving Husband "ART" the Godly Priest of our household and a "Solid Rock" of Strength, Support and Encouragement To Me Always. "I Thank God For You Every Day of My Life Sweetheart More Than You'll Ever Know"

To: Our awesome Daughters and Son Denise C. Bush-Wilson, Roslyn Bush and John A. Bush

God's Joys of my Life

To: Our Grandchildren: Drew, Arthur, Tonoa, Cristina, Joshua, Corey, Courtney, Austin and BJ

God's Loves of My Life

To: Our five Great Grandchildren: Amiah, Karman, Caliyah, Michah and Jason

God's Precious Jewels of My Life

To: Our Precious Parents who made all of us possible through Christ: John and Martha Bush – Eddie and Viola Higgenbotham and Roberson (My Father) and Anna Mae Mczeal

TO: All of my Sisters and Brothers: Dorothy, RJ, Velma, Leatha, Eddie, Richard, Rainey, Gerry, Gail, Don and Annette

In Memory Of Our Baby Brother

Herman Frank Higgenbottham

A TRIBUTE TO OUR MOTHER

Mom has been not just a mother to us but a true inspiration and living testimony of God's love, grace and mercy. Mom has been a Mediator, Intercessor, Confidant, and a Friend. As Matriarch of the Arthar Bush Family, Mom has overcome many obstacles

In her life and through it all, she has always given God the honor, glory, praise and thanksgiving for the good and the bad. The love that she gives to everyone who comes in contact with her is genuine and unprecedented. Our mom's passion for families has made her the surrogate mother and grandmother to so many. Mom takes every opportunity given to minister the word of God in songs, words, and deeds--especially to her children. We are so proud of you, Mom, and all of your achievements and we thank God for blessing us with such a wonderful Mom.

May God Bless You and Keep you, May He always cause His face to shine upon you and Dad and give you Peace forever.

Your, Children,

Dennie, Roz and John "B"

ACKNOWLEDGEMENTS

This book would not have been possible without the help and assistance of the following persons:

Mrs. Colleen Freeman for having faith in me and typing my first manuscript.

Mrs. Arethea Williams for her untiring assistance with both the typing and computer knowledge of manuscript format. Also special thanks to Zachery Williams for his awesome patience with his mom as she worked with me.

A special thanks to Edward and Emilia Marion for their tireless efforts in helping with the reading, rewrites and many suggestions.

Last, but not least, I would like to thank my husband Art for his encouragement, love, patience and understanding during the entire process of my writing God's precious book "To God be the glory Honey: for all He has done for us."

STATEMENT

By

Bishop Devane

I've known Sis. Bush for twelve years and, during that time, I've witnessed how God has used her supernaturally to win lost souls to Christ. Instead of complaining about her physical infirmities, she has always turned it into something to praise God for as Job did ("Though He slay me, yet will I trust in Him - But I will maintain mine own ways before Him") Job 13:15. Her determination to win lost souls for Christ through each physical trial, seems as though it's like fire shut up in her bones rather than the pain that she is physically suffering in her body. In the pass twelve years my wife "Annette" and I have never Heard her ask the question, "Why is God allowing me to suffer this way"? Through it all, her faith has never wavered. It has made her stronger and more determined to do the work for the Lord. When you look at her, all you can see is "God's Master Piece". She is an anointed and praying woman who is led by the Lord. If you ever need someone to reach the Throne of Heaven on your behalf, she'll be right there for you. She lets nothing or no one Hinder her serving God. Her favorite heartbeat confession is "No one or nothing is going to cause me to lose my soul to hell". I am so thankful that God has allowed my family and I to be a part of her life, "For such a time as this". She has been and always will be, a great inspiration in my life. It is a great honor to be called a friend of the Godly woman I call "Sister Fannie Bush."

FORWARD
BY

DR. STEPHEN L. LOWERY

I can't remember the first time I met Fannie Bush or the first time I heard her sing. However, I do well remember that for many years, Fannie was a dedicated woman of God who was able to influence people with her infectious personality and passionate singing for Christ. Though Fannie has a wonderful voice, it was her choice of music and manifest sincerity, as well as the anointing of the holy spirit, that made the diffetrence in her music ministry. Some people can have beautiful voices, but you know that the song does not really come from the heart. With Fannie, not only does the music come from her heart, but also from her experiences.

She lives the relationship to the one of whom she sings.

In 1981, my father, Dr. T. L. Lowery was on a forty day fast seeking direction for his life and felt he was to accept the leadership of a small, troubled work in the Washington, DC area. I owned an electronic corporation in Tennessee and did music ministry on the weekends, but my father asked me to come with him to Washington and build a strong work for God in our nation's capitol. That year, my mother and father, my wife, Janice and our three children, moved to Washington and we have been here ever since. For 26 years (as of November 2007) God has blessed the ministry and today our congregation has more than 3,500 members.

For the first sixteen years at National Church of God, I had the privilege of being Director of Music and Worship Ministries, Director of Radio and Television, Associate Pastor and Ministries Coordinator. In this role as Music Minister, God consistently blessed National Church with wonderfully talented musicians and voices. But, there have been a few that have been of vital importance to the spirituality of the entire ministry. Fannie was a leader in the ministry and could be found making a difference wherever she was at the time.

One of the realities of Fannie's ministry is that you know she lives what she sings. On many occasions, I have spoken of Sister Bush as a 'walking miracle'. My wife and I, along with our choir, music department and congregation would go into fervent prayer during one of many attacks on her body by satan, and we would see God miraculously turn the prognosis around, and heal her body. It was out of this deep faith and trust in God, who was faithful that made Fannie's singing usher in the presence of God. So, when she would sing, "I've got to tell somebody', you knew that she knew what she was talking about.

In 1996, my father was elected back to executive council of the church denomination and moved back to Cleveland, Tennessee. The pastor's council and elders of the National Church of God asked me to take the senior pastor's position, and God continues to bless the ministry. But, it was around that same time that Art and Fannie Bush moved back to Columbia, South Carolina. There have been many times through these last several years that I have missed the friendship and leaership of Art and Fannie. But, what I told them would happen, did happen. Their gifts and talents were just transplanted to another place in God's kingdom, for they have been busy in Columbia, singing, helping, working, leading and organizing. The seeds God plants will always grow and flourish wherever there is good ground.

PREFACE

By Bishop Vincent D. Collins

Welcome to Fannie Bush's initial release "I've Got To Tell Somebody" In this exciting and revolutionizing book it reveals the Love Life and Legacy of a great woman of faith.

The author Fannie Bush not only serves as a member of my local church she is also the spiritual mother of our congregation. God has given her insight to speak a prophetic word for this season. In this book you will find encouragement, hope and a word from God given to a world that seems to be so misguided, where even Christians are discouraged, carrying loads of guilt and burden with all the ills and struggles of our world. The question that many struggle with is "do Christians suffer?" and "1ˢᵗ Peter 2: clearly tells us "To this you were called, because Christ suffered for you, leaving you an example that you should follow in his steps." Our inability to find real solutions to problems is often mirrored in our personal lives, when financial setbacks arise, when our personal dreams are dashed or our children seem bent on self destruction. Then and only then do we ask ourselves in effect, who's in control. We certainly don't feel as if we are. However we long to create order and peace and well being.

What Fannie candidly shares with you in her biography reminds you of the woman with the alabaster box, in spite of all her troubles, tests and tribulations, her rendering was an indication of true surrender to God, His Grace and the Gospel. In this "Life Changing Book," Fannie shares her testimony, life, family experiences and scriptures that will effect and trascend all genders and ages of how to serve God and prevail. "*I've Got To Tell Somebody*" will find it's place as one of the most relevant books you read this year and challenges every person to leave a spiritual inheritance for your family. **This is a must to read.**

INTRODUCTION

By Bishop Doyle Roberts

When we first met in the spring of 2002, I knew that the woman that stood before me was an awesome lady. How? One might ask! I just knew! Sure enough, as time would pass and a Godly relationship built, the evidence of my initial feeling was confirmed.

Over the past five plus years, I have personally witnessed the Holy Spirit's work through the life of Sister Fannie Bush. Let me ask you one question. How can someone with so many different afflictions continue to live a solid life for Christ without complaint? – battle after battle, infirmity after infirmity but live as though none of the season in which they endure stops them from serving Christ. The last thing that we need today is another study from some group of people that study the why and how regarding Christian Maturity. Just giving a testimony of a woman of faith with all of her transparency and her testimony will cheer me on to fight the good fight of faith.

It's amazing in America today that many Christians are growing faint in their fight giving into every *whelm* that would keep them from fully recognizing their full potential as to what God has planned for them. Not with this woman of God! She has made up in her mind that she will serve the Lord and that her source is in Him (Jesus Christ) in whom she live, move, breathe and have her being. Evidence in her book is her strength in realizing the power of the scripture. Over and over she places emphasis on the word of God as she quotes scripture that brings her life and strength necessary to fight every circumstance that comes her way. In just a short time of watching this precious saint of

God's faith walk, she has spoken volumes of wisdom into my life by watching her endurance to keep going in Christ.

Every day there are decisions that people make that directly affect their lives either positively or negatively. One of the most important decisions from the Author's perspective was to become a born again believer - a Christian.

This book takes a look at the life of Fannie Bush, an African American girl dealing with poverty, prejudices and infirmities from age three to woman-hood. She also share the awesome and happy times of marrying the man of her dreams, having children, grandchildren, great-grandchildren to now a woman in her seventies who has examined her life in the concept of making the wrong and right decisions and how they affected her life. Fannie's book is intertwined with words of wisdom that can help the reader candidly learn from her life that could prevent someone from making wrong choices but at the same time, be able to quickly learn the most important factor of her life that brought the much needed stability.... a relationship with the Lord Jesus Christ.

Her book begins by describing various aspects of her childhood relating to different issues of life that are honest renditions dealing with her own struggles of life and how she overcame each. She is carefully transparent and even sometimes radical in describing some of the experiences that she had while on this journey between the flesh (natural woman) and the spirit. Her natural man says one thing and her spirit says another. The question is who will win?

Sister Fannie's desire is to influence the reader that regardless of what life may deal out to you, there is the opportunity to pass the test or to fail. Her stance is simple but yet profound ...that without Christ, it is impossible to pass the test. I thank God for her candidness relating to her position in various battles that she has fought to even the record of her thoughts and how she, through many wrongs at a young age, turned to make the right decisions and how it affected her outcome regarding the record of her life experiences to this point.

We can only imagine what the outcome would have been without the influence of Christ and the Holy Spirit in her life encouraging her not to give up! That's why she must "TELL SOMEBODY" because I believe that if just one reader grabs a hold of this precious woman's stance regarding her life, it will be worth the battle of her writing her life's testimony to share with the world.

Table of Contents

-THIS IS MY STORY-

I was born in a very small town in Lake Arthur, Louisiana. My mother and stepfather raised eight children—four boys and four girls. Our parents were godly parents and raised us in the church. As a matter of fact, we were in church every time the doors opened for Sunday school, church services, Bible training, choir rehearsal, or any other special program. We were there during the school months when, regardless of the weather, we had to walk two to three miles to school. Simply put, there was no excuse to skip church. I also remember as a little girl how much I loved to sing church songs. My mom realized that God had given me a gift to sing at the age of five. From that time on, all I wanted to do was to sing for Jesus.

To me, my mother was blessed with the most beautiful voice in the world. I can remember every morning during the winter, she would get up around 5:00 a.m. and begin her daily routine while singing, "Oh How I Love Jesus." She would sing as she was putting wood in the old potbelly stove located between our living room and dining room. That old stove would heat up the whole house before we got out of bed.

She would continue to sing as she cooked oatmeal, grits, or cream of wheat for our breakfast before sending us off to school. I am sure she would continue singing even more beautifully after she was blessed with the privilege of sending us to school.

During that time, we had no idea what a bathroom was. Instead, we had an outdoor toilet, commonly known as an "Out House" in the back yard, which consisted of a little house with a door for privacy and a hole dug into the earth. There was a wooden top placed over the hole that was dug into the earth, large enough for us to sit on. This wooden top was called our toilet seat. Praise God!

As a child, I was always afraid that I would fall into the hole, so I would hold on for dear life to avoid falling through it. I can vividly remember the maggots that lived in the hole and fed off of the feces and urine.

We didn't have a washing machine or a bathtub either. We had what we called a (wash tub). When Mom washed our clothes in the tub, she would heat buckets of water from our outdoor pump on our iron stove and fill the tub with water. She used what we called a washing board to wash our clothes. When we bathed, she would also heat water on our iron stove and fill the tub for us to bathe. My sister Leatha and I would bathe together since we were the youngest girls. We always had so much fun in the bathtub that our mom would have to insist that we get out of the water. We also didn't know what an electric iron was. So we would iron our clothes with what we called a hot iron, which we heated on the top of the iron stove she used for cooking.

Even with all of these things that we would consider inconveniences today, we were a happy family. Even during those days, I remember being a sickly child. However, I was too young to understand why God was allowing these things to happen to me. Before I was old enough to attend school, I developed a condition called Rickets. This disease would cripple little babies from about two years old to the ages of three to five years.

But God had another plan for my life. Even though I did not know how to pray, my mom and step father, who were prayer warriors, touched and agreed on my behalf, according to God's word in Matthew 18:19–20. "Again, I tell you that if two of you on earth agree about anything you ask for, it will be done for you by my Father in Heaven. For where two or three come together in my name, there am I in the midst of them." Praise God! By the time I was six years old, I was more than able to attend my first school year without missing a day.

My sisters, Dorothy, Velma and Leatha, told me that during the years I couldn't walk, I was a regular "Dennis the Menace". I would do all kinds of mischievous things that caused them to be chastised. They also thought I was the funniest little thing they had ever seen. No matter how I felt, I could always make them laugh. They said I didn't cry much, but when I did, they understood why.

One of the times I loved most was when my sisters would take me for walks to play with the other kids. Dorothy would always carry me on her right hip, and the adults, especially the grandmothers, would be sitting on their front porches, watching the children from the neighborhood play on the street. They never worried about us getting hit by a car because there were no car owners on our side of town. We literally had to walk wherever we wanted to go in town. The adults always warned my sister Dorothy that if she continued to carry me on her hips, one of her hips would develop lower than the other. She continued to do so, and today she walks with one hip slightly lower than the other. Every time I see her, I just want to throw my arms around her and tell her how much I love her. "THAT'S WHY I'VE GOT TO TELL SOMEBODY".

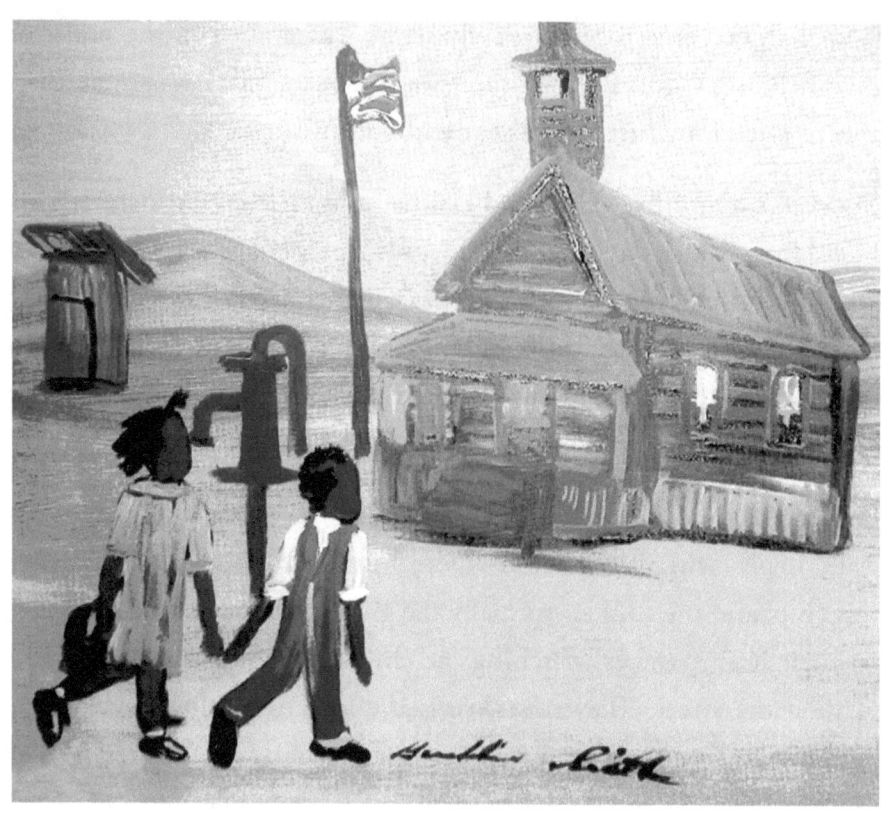

The Toliet- The Water Pump- The School Building

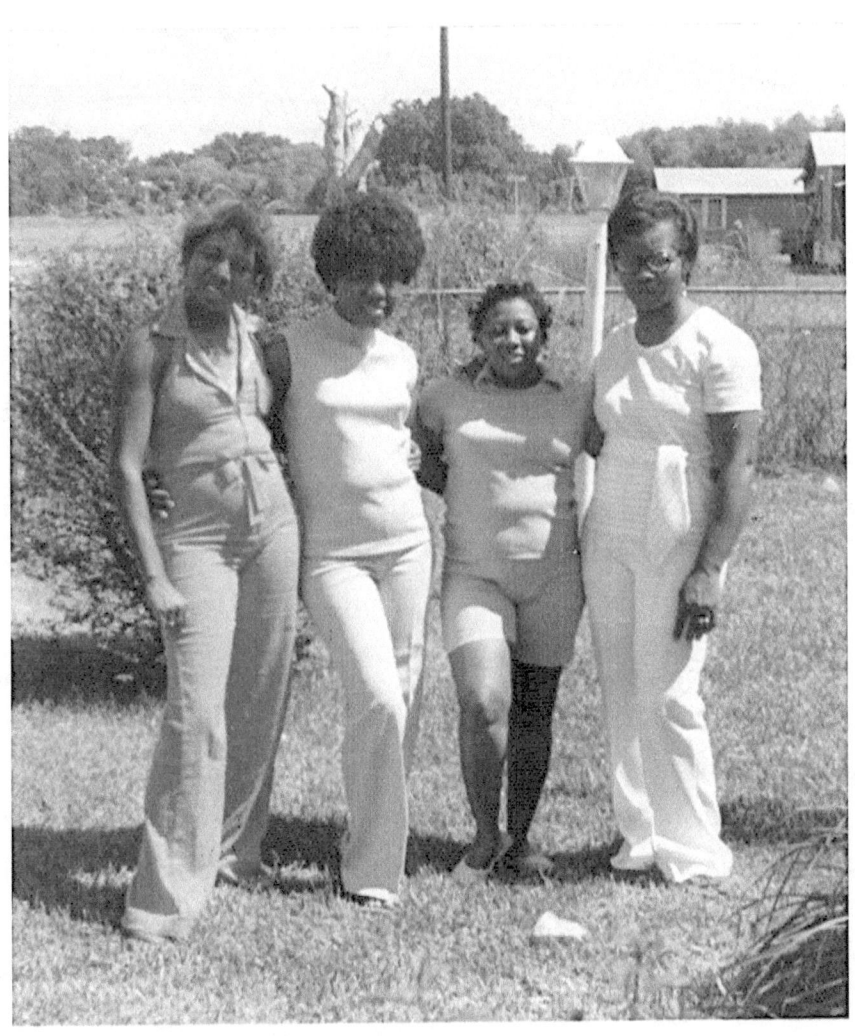

Fannie with her sisters: Dorothy, Leatha and Velma

-GROWING UP-

As I matured, it occurred to me that I loved Jesus but did not understand God's Holy Word, the Bible. I made excuses for my ignorance of God's word because I did not understand thous, trespasses, names of people, tribes, and so much more. It became more frustrating when I began to notice that even younger people knew more about the Bible than me. I was ashamed to ask questions or let them know that I was ignorant of God's Word. I thought that as long as I attended church regularly and sang in the choir, then surely I was on my way to Heaven.

All my life, I grew up in the church according to my stepfather and mother's standards. I will love them with all my heart as long as I live for raising me in the admonition of Christ Jesus. Every day of my life, I praise God for having them plant the seed in my heart so that one day someone would come into my life and water it and God would give me the increase with love overflowing for Him as long as I live. At seventeen years of age, I began noticing young people my age going places, dancing, drinking, smoking, and talking about girlfriends and boyfriends. And, like most young girls, I wanted to experience all of those things as well. But our parents, especially our mom, watched over us girls like a mother bear watches over her cubs—touch them in front of her and you may not see another day.

Being the youngest of four girls, it became clear to me by the time I was in the eleventh grade that my mother was well versed on the behavioral pattern of girls my age. My junior and senior proms validated this belief. I was allowed to have a date, but my mother, and several mothers of the same mindset, would walk a distance behind us. At the prom, they would sit in chairs along the walls of the prom and have fun (I think). When the prom ended, they would follow us home, making sure that there was no, as they phrased it during that time, hanky panky going on.

Upon completing the twelfth grade, I was allowed to go to the prom unescorted by my mom. However, when my date and I came around the corner to our home, my mom and stepfather were leisurely swinging away on the front porch swing, waiting for me. With our options limited, my date and I had no choice but to give each other a peck on the cheek and say good night.

If you think that was rough, when I was sixteen, I had a crush on a young man of seventeen who had given me a love note. Somehow, the note must have fallen out of my books and onto our dining room table, where we did our homework every day. Well, of all people, my mom found it! The note told of how much he enjoyed kissing me on my cheek. My mom was fit to be tired. Translation: She was furious! I'd never seen her so angry with me before. After she finished lecturing me on the ways of the world, I just burst out crying, and then I asked her, "Does that mean I'm pregnant?"

I thought that she would never stop laughing. I believe, to her, that was enough punishment for me. "THAT'S WHY I'VE GOT TO TELL SOMEBODY."

-MEETING THE MAN OF MY DREAMS THROUGH CHRIST-

After graduation, I was off to McNeese State College in Lake Charles, Louisiana. My mother insisted that I live with my sister. I loved that! My only regret was that I was unable to live in the dormitory with my two best friends from high school. Once I realized that my parents were no longer in control of my life, I hardly ever went to church. I began to thoroughly enjoy the life of a single female.

While in college, I went to class every day and worked nights at an ice cream stand beside a movie theater. One night, a young man came up to my window to order an ice cream cone. He had the bluest eyes I had ever seen. He was kind of cute and the perfect height—about six feet three inches tall. I'd always said that my husband would be tall, dark, and handsome. However, at that point, I immediately realized that he'd filled all of the qualifications, but he had blue eyes and he wasn't dark (black).

When he approached my window, he said, "If I tell you your name, would you give me my cone free?"

I just laughed.

Then he said, "Your name is Fannie B. McZeal."

I was in shock.

He finally confessed that he and my sister, Dorothy, were in the same class, studying for their GED certificates. He said he saw Dorothy standing by a soda machine during their class break and he approached her and offered to buy her a soda. She quickly responded and very proudly said that she was married. I interrupted him right then because he was getting on my last nerve. Besides, there was a long line of servicemen behind him who were looking at him kind of rough.

I tried to tell him in a nice way that I'd never seen him before in my life, but he said, "I really did talk with your sister, and she told me all about you. I asked her if she had a sister at home who looked like her, and she told me about you."

About a week later, he called me for a date to the movies, and I accepted immediately, but I thought to myself, *why did I do that?*

It was about that time I realized in my heart that God does work things out for our benefit.

When our date ended at my sister's front door, he asked me for a kiss good night. I politely told him my mom taught me never to kiss a boy on the first date. At that point, he looked down at me and said, "Girl, I'm going to marry you one day."

"Oh no, no, no you are not my type because you are white," was my response.

He then said, "I'm not white. My father is white."

And that's when I reminded him that God's word tells us "thou shall not lie".

Then he said, "But my mother is Indian."

To be smart, I told him, "I love my men black."

Obviously that didn't offend him at all, and I was glad it didn't because I sort of liked him a lot.

However, my goal was to finish college with a nursing degree. Then, if I met someone, preferably a doctor, I'd fall in love, and maybe after a year or two, we would get married. Although it was a great plan, after several months of Art and I dating, the spirit of lust overwhelmed our ability to remember our upbringing at home—most of all, what Jesus said in I Corinthians 6:13, "The body is not made for sexual immorality, but for the Lord, and the Lord for the body."

By the time I'd reached my sophomore year in college, I was with child. Both of us had to seek God's face and ask Him to forgive us of our sins and cleanse us from all unrighteousness, according to His word in I John 1:9, and that is, "If we confess our sins, God is faithful and just to forgive us of our sins and cleanse us from all unrighteousness."

Knowing that we loved each other, we were married in my sister Dorothy's home. "THAT'S WHY I'VE GOT TO TELL SOMEBODY."

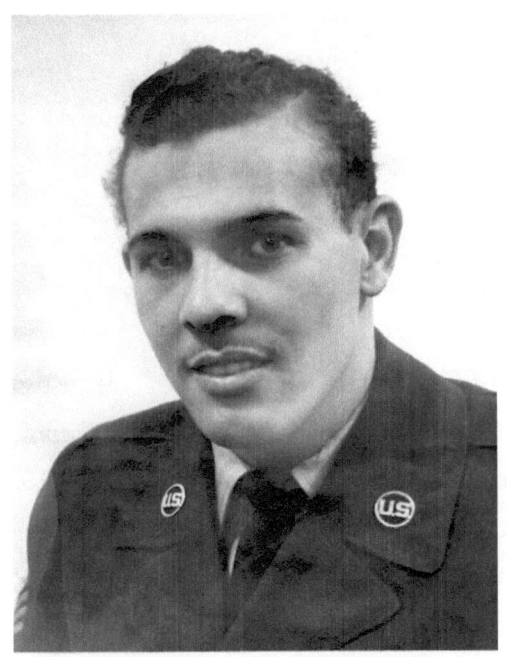

Fannie's Husband Art Bush

-GOD'S GRACE-

After getting married, I dropped out of college due to our financial situation, and I became a stay-at-home mom. I was eighteen years old. I think, at that point in our lives, we were too young to know the real meaning of love. However, I can truly say that we've been victorious through the blood of Jesus Christ. Today, we stand steadfast and immovable on I John 1:9. Praise God!

God has blessed us with two wonderful children, nine grandchildren, and five great-grandchildren. We have claimed them all for the Kingdom of Heaven as we have prayed and interceded for them every day. We have constantly stood on God's Holy Word in Proverbs 11:21, "The seed of the righteous shall be delivered."

Our children are our seeds, and my husband and I are the righteousness of God almighty. For the past fifty one years, we've experienced what true love really means between a man and a woman of God because of the love of our Lord and Savior, Jesus Christ.

The first year of our marriage wasn't easy...especially for our little baby Denise, whom we lovingly call Dennie. When she was a baby, my husband, Art, was in the Air Force as Airman First Class. We lived in a little house, which had one small room with a double bed, a sofa, our baby's bed, and a small kitchen. Even though we had a toilet connected to the house, we had to open the side door of the house, step down two steps, and then go up two steps into the toilet. Praise God! Inside the little room was a real commode that flushed—*hallelujah*! Just like the Jeffersons, "WE WERE MOVING ON UP."

The house was infested with roaches. We had no knowledge of covering ourselves and our baby with the Blood of Jesus. But the God of our childhood kept us through it all.

Our first income tax statement was about $1,948 that first year, including an $81-per-month allotment check provided to military wives based on their husband's rank—but God kept us. On top of it all, we were living in a time when the slogan in America was as real as we were: "If you are black, step back."

We were struggling to survive in a world of discrimination. Most of the time, all we had were each other. We had no money to travel and visit our families, especially my husband who was from Columbia, South Carolina. At least we were stationed in Louisiana, which was my home state. Again, God kept us.

The next two years, my husband, whom I lovingly call Sweetheart, made Airman Second Class. Then we had to start getting ready for our bundle of joy, our son John, whom I lovingly call, John B. A month after John's birth, my husband was shipped to Germany; six months later, we were on our way to Germany.

We lived in Ramstein Germany, for about four and half years. It was during that time that I realized our lives were empty. God was no longer in our lives. Then one night in the summer months, we heard songs of praise unto God from the building next door. They were having prayer service. So Art and I decided to go to the next prayer service and ask if we could join them. They welcomed us with opened arms. Soon the group grew so large that we had to rent the German church nearby to have service, but I still did not honor God as I should have. I had given up on God, but God had not given up on me. Needless to say, we were eventually sent back to the United States. Our assignment was Wichita Falls, Texas. It was there that I returned to college. I put all of myself into my studies and spent very little time with God. By the time we left Texas, we were full of the world. Our next assignment was Andrews Air Force Base in Suitland, Maryland. "THAT'S WHY I'VE GOT TO TELL SOMEBODY."

-GOD'S MERCY-

We found an apartment in Southeast Washington, DC, which was not too far from the air base. We also found a church right around the corner called, Emmanuel Baptist Church. Since my husband and I was both raised Baptist, we started attending Emmanuel and eventually joined. Once again, it was the music that had drawn me in. I immediately joined the choir because they were seeking choir members.

Later on, after the choir director heard my voice leading the choir several times, she asked me to join the all women singing group, The Friendly Gospel Singers. That's when I realized, once again, that God was real.

Emmanuel Baptist Church soon became our home away from home, and I loved the members there dearly. They will always be an extension of our family of God. I love them more today than yesterday. At Emmanuel, the word of God became real to me like never before. "THAT'S WHY I'VE GOT TO TELL SOMEBODY."

-GOD'S SALVATION-

Our family church in Lake Arthur, Louisiana, was Antioch Baptist Church. My mother was determined to lead us (whether we appreciated it or not) to Jesus Christ our Lord and Savior so that, when we got older, we would not depart from Him. There was one scripture my mother taught us that I will never forget—Romans 10:13, "Whosoever shall call on the name of Jesus, shall be saved."

When my mother taught me that scripture, I knew then that I belonged to Jesus. I never knew anyone who would call on the name of Jesus as often as my mother did. The one thing that she told us every day was to remember this, if you don't remember anything else in your life: "Jesus will never leave you or forsake you."

She also taught us how to lean and depend upon Jesus, and to always remember, without a doubt, that God's grace is sufficient for us and His mercy is everlasting.

I'd lived in Lake Arthur all my life, in a town where my parents could barely make a living for us. I finished high school, and I was the only one to attend college. I married a military man, and we've been married for fifty-one years…praise God! God has given us two wonderful children, and He has blessed me to be able to travel to amazing places, such as Jerusalem, Egypt, Guatemala, Germany, France, and Jamaica to minister the Gospel of Jesus Christ in music, to sail the sea of Galilee, to be baptized in the River Jordan where Jesus was baptized, to walk the Via Dolorosa where Jesus carried His cross all the way up to Golgotha where He was crucified for our sins, and to walk in the tomb where our Savior was buried and rose from the dead!

In my job with the Federal Government in Washington, DC, I had the opportunity to travel extensively throughout the United States. Through all of my travels, God kept me just as my mother had said He would, and I found out for myself that, according to Hebrews 13:8, "He's the same yesterday, today, and forever."

That is why I can truly testify to the world today that God has proven Himself to me over and over again. This is the same truth my mother passed on to me about Jesus when I was a child. Many years ago, she taught me what I call precious: words of life about Jesus. Those words are, "When your father and mother are gone, call Jesus. He's your father, your mother, your sister, your brother, your husband, your friend your all in all. When you don't know whom to call on, call Jesus - When you feel like you don't have a friend, call Jesus - When Satan and his principalities and powers, rulers of darkness and spiritual weakness in high places, come against you, call Jesus."

"Before He allows His child to be chewed up and spit out by this world, Jesus will be right there in the midst of it all. He will give you the strength you need to shake that old devil off and crush his head under your feet." II Corinthians 12:9–10 says, "And He said unto me, my grace is sufficient for thee—for my strength is made perfect in weakness. Most gladly therefore will I rather glory in my infirmities, that the power of Christ may rest upon me. Therefore I take pleasure in my infirmities, my reproaches, in necessities, in persecutions, in distresses for Christ's sake; for when I am weak, then I am strong." "THAT'S WHY I'VE GOT TO TELL SOMEBODY."

-FALLING FROM GRACE-

Several years later, my husband and I began to realize how dangerous it was for our children to live in the city. We decided to build our home in the small town of Upper Marlboro, Maryland, in the gated community of Marlboro Meadows. We lived there until both of our children graduated from high school. Then we decided to build another home in Fort Washington, Maryland, with close access to Washington, Maryland, and Virginia.

By this time, I had become very successful working for the Federal Government. God began to bless my husband even more with promotion after promotion. Most of all, He began to open our hearts and pour more love in our hearts for each other like never before. It's a love that reminds us every day of Matthew 19:6, "Whom God has joined together, let no man put asunder."

We had our health and strength, and we thought we had our right minds. However, we never stopped to take time to think about where this abundant love was coming from. We never took the time to seek God's will for our lives and seek His face. In other words, we never stopped to remember where our help came from. We sincerely believed in our hearts that we could say "Well God, you've done your part; we can take it from here. We'll call on you when, and if, we need you again."

We were a two-car family, had wonderful avenues of entertainment (parties, movies, travel, etc), and a church we attended at our convenience. I was still singing in the choir and with The Friendly Gospel Singers and my husband was still singing in the men's choir. Most of the time, we only attended church when we had to sing or on Communion Sunday, drinking damnation to our souls. I Corinthians 11:29 tells us, "For anyone who drinks without recognizing the body of the Lord eats and drinks judgment on himself." Even though God so graciously blessed us, we gave to Him whatever we chose to give. We did not want to hear anyone talk about tithing. But I thank our God for forgiving us. "THAT'S WHY I'VE GOT TO TELL SOMEBODY."

-FROM THE PIT TO THE PALACE-

My husband and I both came from large families. My husband's father and mother had thirteen children, plus two children who they raised from infancy due to an untimely death of one of his sisters. And as I mentioned earlier, my mom and stepfather had eight children. My father had two daughters and two sons. I love every one of them with all my heart with a love that the devil and all his principalities, powers, rulers of darkness, and spiritual wickedness in high places can destroy. Our parents had so much love and respect for each other. They truly exhibited that love (godly love) for each other as long as I can remember. They became perfect examples for all of us.

God has been so good to all of us. Out of all of my husband's brothers and sisters, only five are living—six counting our niece, Betty, whose mother died when she was a tiny baby. One of my brothers, Herman, was murdered in Washington, DC. All of my other brothers and sisters to this date, October 15, 2007, are still alive.

When I remember how our parents had to struggle every day taking care of their families and think about where God has brought Art and I today from meager backgrounds with strong godly parents, I can truly proclaim that God has brought us from the "Pit To The Palace." "THAT'S WHY I'VE GOT TO TELL SOMEBODY."

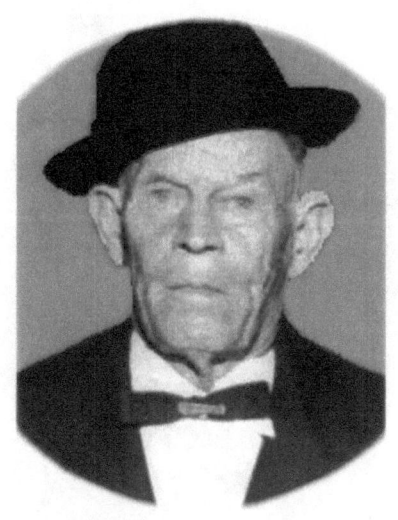

Art's Father, John Westly Bush

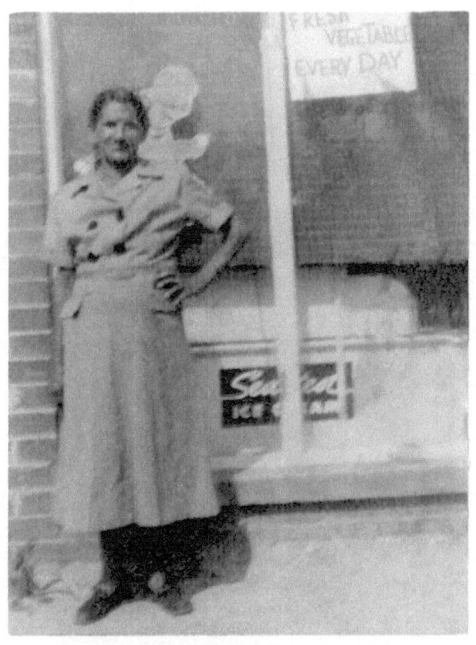

Art's Mother, Martha Bush

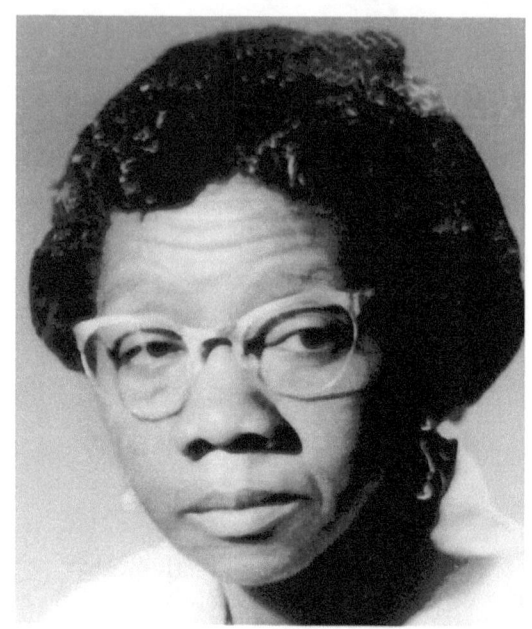

Fannie's Mother, Viola Higgenbotham

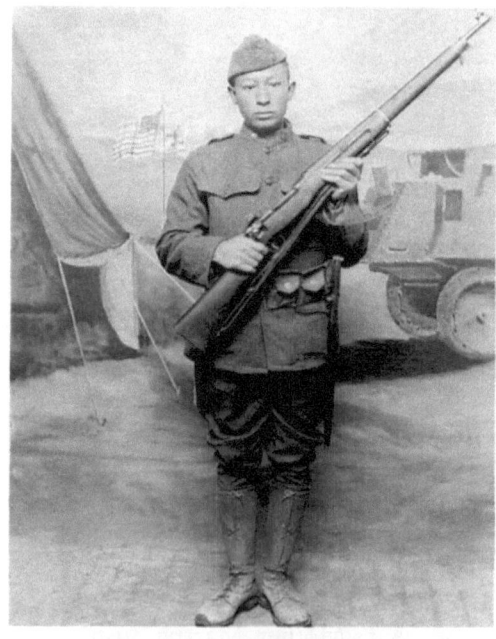

Fannie's Stepfather, Eddie Higgenbotham

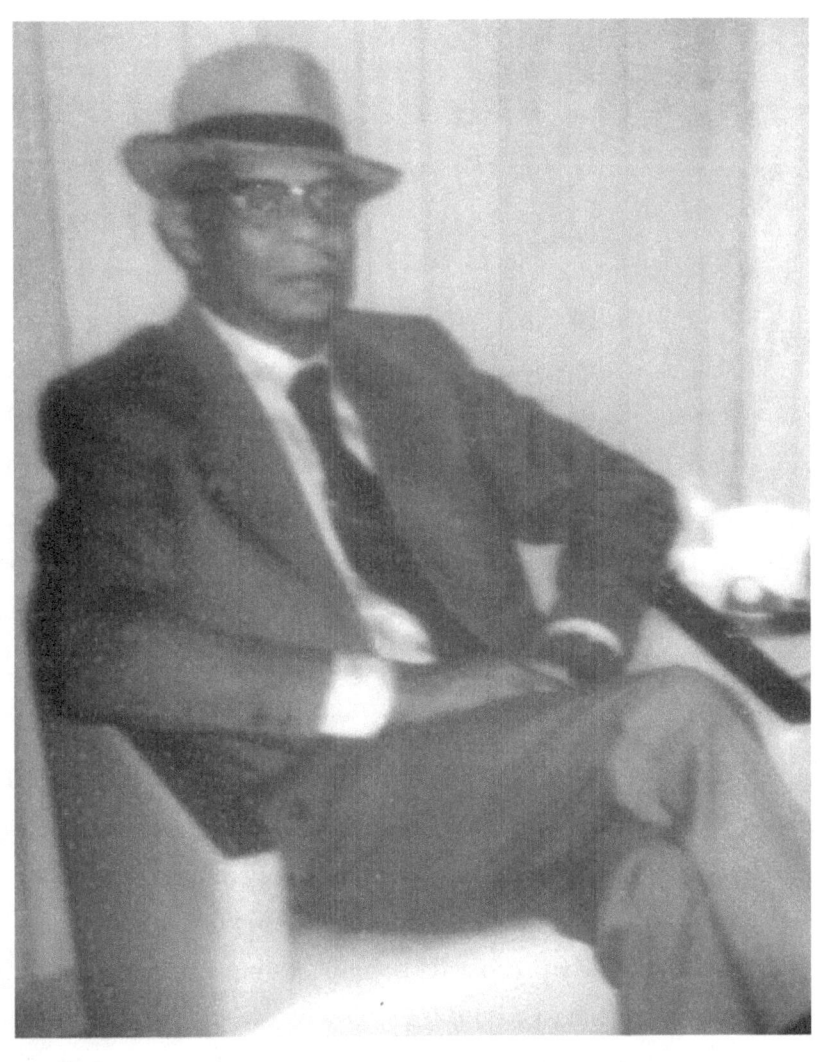

Fannie's Father, Robinson McZeal

-CHOSEN BY GOD-

My mom called me a "Tom-Boy" after I learned how to walk. I thought there was nothing I couldn't do. I would challenge my brothers and sisters to prove to them that I could do anything they could. My mom would always remind me that little girls should not fight little boys, and especially not their sisters. I remember insisting on playing football, baseball and boxing with my brothers. I allowed them to take me by my feet and swing me around in the air then let me go to see which one would catch me. It was rough, but I sure did enjoy my brothers, RJ, Eddie, Richard, and Herman.

We lived in an area where the baseball field was between our home and the lake. My mom and stepfather would allow us to go there as long as our older sisters or brothers were with us. I'd wanted to learn how to swim forever, it seemed. When I was seven years old, we were playing around in the lake. My brother RJ convinced me that if I would stand on my head in the lake, I would learn how to swim. I almost drowned that day. I also remember when he told me to fall into his arms from our high porch banister, promising me faithfully that he would catch me. Well he didn't. I wound up with a broken arm.

My brother Eddie and I were so close, and we always got into trouble together (partners in crime). One day I told my stepfather the truth about something Eddie had done, and he was chastised. A few days later, Eddie saw me sitting on our front porch steps eating watermelon, and he came from behind me and stuck a pair of scissors into the top of my head. But I love my brother more today than yesterday.

My best friend got angry with me because she lost the hopscotch game we always played together. She hit me in the head right around my eyebrow, cutting it open. The scar remains there today, but I love her more today than yesterday.

One year we were renovating our home, and there was a stack of lumber piled up in our yard. The builders had warned us not to play around the lumber. However, after a couple of days, I was bored and decided to play around the lumber. As you might guess, some of the stack fell on top of me. Well, I didn't walk for a long time, but I couldn't sit for a little while either.

When our daughter Dennie was about two years old, I started getting sick and the doctors could not find out what was wrong. After two months in the hospital, they discovered that my blood count was unfavorable, and they began giving me shots in my hips and arms three times a day. During the third month, after all the testing was done, I was told that I had leukemia. However, I knew that my mom and step dad were interceding for me, and God healed me.

Finally, about the fourth month, when man had done what man could do, I was released from the hospital with a certain kind of medication that I stopped taking as soon as I got home. I had not seen my baby, Dennie, for four months and remember so well how hurt I was when I arrived at my mother's house to take her home and she didn't know who I was. She actually ran away from me, and all I could do was cry. However, it wasn't long before she remembered me.

For a short time, I was fine and continued to live straddling the fence. Then one day I began to have terrible pains in my back. They were pains like I'd never felt before in my life. For three years, the pain became unbearable no matter what kind of treatment the doctors would recommend. Finally, in 1971, the only alternative was surgery. Even then, I never stopped to thank God for healing my body and delivering me from evil like He had done so many times before.

Although the operation was a success, the pain returned in the same area in 1974. The doctors told me that two of the upper vertebras in my neck were ruptured and all the trigger point injections were not helping. Once again, I was in surgery. This time, God blessed me and He healed my back completely. However, I was still walking in darkness and was too carnal-minded to realize that it was God's grace and mercy that kept me. Praise your name, Lord Jesus!

But we still had not totally committed our lives completely to God, but what a rude awakening we received in October of 1983. "THAT'S WHY I'VE GOT TO TELL SOMEBODY."

-MY DELIVERANCE-

I remember October of 1983 very well. I visited my doctor's office for a routine physical, and after he'd completed my exam, he informed me that everything was fine. However, for some reason (I now know that it was the hands of Jesus), I continued to feel under my arms, and eventually felt a small nodule about the size of a pencil point. I immediately stopped the doctor from washing his hands and informed him that I felt something under my arm. He checked the area and said that he didn't like the shape of the pimple that he felt, and he requested a mammogram of my breast. Three days later, the radiologist called to inform me that he needed to redo the mammogram of my left breast. Of course, I was shocked. This could not be happening to me. I never thought of praying...nor did my husband, not for a second. Three days later, I was in the hospital having biopsies done on both my breasts. When the doctors informed my husband and I that there was cancer in my left breast, it was like delivering a death sentence. Three days later, I lost my left breast to cancer.

However, there's a moment that I will never forget at that time in my life when God gave me peace. I remember the night before my surgery, when the doctor came into my room to talk to my husband about the surgery. He came into my room holding a medical book with the picture of what my body would look like after my surgery and for the rest of my life. He proceeded to show the picture to my husband. My husband looked at the picture very carefully. He then looked up at the surgeon and said, "Doctor, I always thought two were too many, anyway." At that point, the three of us started laughing with tears coming down our faces.

The doctor looked at us and said, "Sometimes I wonder why bad things happen to wonderful people like you," and he walked out of the room with those same tears running down his face.

Later on, as I continued to visit the doctor for checkups, God gave me the opportunity to minister to that same doctor through His holy word. We remain friends today, and my husband and I dearly love him and we look forward to seeing him in Heaven someday. Once again, God proved to us that He will give us peace in the midst of a storm. Satan was a liar in the name of Jesus. But God kept me. That's why "I'VE GOT TO TELL SOMEBODY."

During my two weeks of recuperation. I saw the surgeon again. I knew that there might be some hard decisions for me to make in regard to chemotherapy or radiation treatments. However, I believe that I'd already decided not to have any treatments. And at that moment, I remembered my mom's words of wisdom: "Baby, when you don't know what to do, call on Jesus."

So I called on Jesus, and I knew that everything would be fine.

The day finally came when I had to get the results from my doctor as to what the next steps would be. That morning, I was trying to dress, but my left arm was so sore I could hardly raise it up. I kept calling for my husband to help me dress, but he didn't answer me. Then I started crying. Suddenly, he came out of the bathroom, and I asked him, "Why didn't you come when I called?"

He said to me, "Honey, you won't have to have chemotherapy or radiation."

I responded like a doubting Thomas. "Honey, don't play with me that way."

And then he said, "Honey, I'm not playing. I just finished praying to God, asking Him to deliver you from taking chemo or radiation."

So we touched and agreed according to Matthew 18:19, "Again, I tell you that if two of you on earth agree about anything you ask for, it will be done for you by your Father in heaven."

When the doctor saw us that day, he had the pathologist's report in his hand and he said to me, "Mrs. Bush, go home and live! You don't need any treatment. We got it all." *Hallelujah!*

Oh how we praised God that day. We knew, without a doubt, that God kept us, and "THAT'S WHY I'VE GOT TO TELL SOMEBODY."

-THE DIVINE REVELATION OF JESUS-

I remember very well the Friday night I came from the hospital. Some of our family members had come from my husband's home, Columbia, South Carolina. They were all downstairs, laughing and talking, and waiting to see me. I remember how they would come up to see me two at a time. After the last person had gone down the stairs, I began to cry out to the Lord as best I knew how and said, "Lord, everybody downstairs is laughing and full of life, and all I can feel is the pain of death."

All of a sudden, I began to feel warmth at the foot of my bed, and I knew immediately that it wasn't evil. I could feel it in my spirit, and I knew at that moment it was the presence of Jesus.

He said to me, "Choose ye this day whom you will serve…you can't serve me and Satan too. You can choose me and live or choose Satan and die."

I can remember saying to Jesus, "Lord, if you let me live, I'll go where you want me to go, I'll do what you want me to do, and I'll say what you want me say, as long as I live."

I've been running for Jesus every since. However, my husband was still not completely sold out to Christ and was still straddling the fence and living in both worlds. The Holy Spirit would always remind me in I Corinthians 7:14, "For the unbelieving husband has been sanctified through his wife, and an unbelieving wife has been sanctified through her believing husband." So, I began to study the word of God every day as though each day was my last ever interceding for my husband. "THAT'S WHY I'VE GOT TO TELL SOMEBODY."

-MY CHOIR DIRECTOR -

One of the most precious memories that I praise God for is the day after surgery when Gerry, my choir director, came to visit and pray for me in the hospital. I believe she was aware of my lifestyle and tried to witness to me at times, but I just ignored the message of life she was trying to convey to me. She came over to my bed with the Bible and another book entitled, *The "B" Attitudes* and suggested that I read them…especially the Bible. Then the next thing I knew, I had knocked the books out of her hands and to the floor. I immediately began to cry like a baby, because I was too ashamed to tell her that I had very little knowledge of the Bible.

Gerry picked up the Bible and The *"B" Attitudes* book and placed them on my bed table. Early the next morning, I woke up with so much pain that I could hardly breathe. However, when my vision cleared, I was staring directly at the table where Gerry had placed the books the day before. I reached out for those precious jewels of life, and for the first time in my life, I could read the Bible without the fear of not being able to understand the height and depth of God's love for me. Did I understand it all then? No. But God, at that very hour, had gotten my attention forever. It was that very day that I decided that I would stand forever on II Timothy 2:15 "Do your best to present yourself to God as one approved, a workman who does not need to be ashamed and who correctly handles the word of truth."

I was in the hospital for seven days, and the more I studied God's word, the more the pain lessened. I knew without a doubt that the hands of Jesus, and Jesus alone, had touched me. My Jehovah Rapha, my healer. From that day forward, I began to study God's word day and night, especially when the spirit of the Lord would wake me up at 1:15 a.m. every morning for approximately six months. He would lead me down the hall to our kitchen and taught me literally everything I know about God's Holy Word, from cover to cover. Amen!

The Lord revealed Himself to me in His power and might, from that moment on, letting me know that I am His own…a chosen child of God. My confession every day in my heart comes from Psalms 12:1–8, "I will lift my eyes unto the hill from whence cometh my help my help cometh from the Lord, which made the Heaven and the Earth. He will not suffer my feet to be moved He that keepth Israel shall neither slumber nor sleep. The Lord is my keeper; the Lord is my shade upon my right hand, the sun shall not spite thee by day nor the moon by night. The Lord shall preserve thee from all evil; He shall preserve thy going out and thy coming in from this time forth and even for evermore." "THAT'S WHY I'VE GOT TO TELL SOMEBODY."

-CHOSEN FOR GOD'S GLORY-

O nce I became a spirit-filled child of God and confessed Jesus as my Lord and Savior, I quickly realized that the battle had just begun, in the form of spiritual warfare. I discerned in my spirit that there was a greater power in me (God's Holy Spirit) than he who is in the world. Also, my God told me in Isaiah 54:17, "No weapon forged against you will prevail, and you will refute every tongue that accuses you."

Therefore, I knew without a doubt that the victory would always be mine when the battle was the Lord's. Praise the mighty name of Jesus!

For three years, I continued to have unfavorable reports regarding my right breast with each mammogram.

In 1988, as I grew stronger in the Lord and the power of His might, I received my last unfavorable report from my doctor. I was told that I had to wait another year for my next X-ray. Well, on my way from the doctor's office, the Spirit of the Lord rose up inside me, and I began to scream out loud in my car, "You're a liar, Satan, and the truth is not in you! I plead the blood of Jesus against you. You are a defeated foe, and I am a child of the Most High God, because He tells me in I John 4:4 'Ye are of God, little children, and have overcome them: because greater is he that is in you; than he that is in the world.'"

All of a sudden, I felt a freedom that could only come from God and God alone.

As soon as I got home, I immediately called my pastor to ask to see him right away.

"Yes, of course, Sister Bush," he said.

When I arrived, he called in two assistant pastors, and they laid hands on me and touched Heaven on my behalf as I surrendered to the Holy Spirit. When I left the church that day, I knew that I would never be the same again…that I would be walking in a greater anointing from that day forward. As soon as I returned home, I laid prostrated on our living room floor (face down) before God. As I laid there before Him, I heard these words in my spirit: "Didn't I tell you in Matthew 5:29 'If your right eye offend you and causes you to sin, gouge it out and throw it away. It is better for you to lose one part of your body than for your whole body to be thrown into hell'?"

This was confirmation from God for me. It was just days before I'd told my husband that I was tired of this demon of cancer tormenting my life and interfering with my work for the Lord and my family. If I had to, I would opt to have my right breast removed. The two of us touched and agreed that same day in Jesus' name.

I decided to have my right breast removed in November of 1988. Once again, the doctor confirmed that I did not have to have chemotherapy or radiation treatments. "Hallelujah," I proclaimed in Jesus' name

And I remembered God's words vividly, according to Psalms 37:4, "Delight yourself in the Lord, and He will give you the desires of your heart." Oh how I delight myself in my God.

I also began to stand on God's precious words of life spoken into my spirit, such as:

- Job 5:26—"I shall go to my grave in a full age like as a shock of corn cometh in it's season."

- Psalms 90:10—"The days of my years are three score and ten or four score and ten, if we have the strength."

- Psalms 34:19—"Many are the afflictions of the righteous but the Lord delivers them out of them all."

- Psalms 103:5—"He promised to satisfy my mouth with good things so that my youth is renewed like the eagles."

- 1 Peter 2:24—"Who His own self bore my sins in His own body on the tree that I being dead to sin should live unto righteousness, by whose stripes, I was healed."

I call I Peter 2:24, "My Smoking Gun" against Satan. I am determined to stand victorious in God's word as long as I live.

I began to realize that God had a plan for my life before I was conceived in my mother's womb. He knew that because of my sins, I would have to suffer. But through my suffering, I would surrender my life to Him so that He could use me to be a witness for Him. Romans 3:23 says "For all have sinned and fallen short of the glory of God."

Through my music ministry, I am using the anointed voice He has given me; counseling and leading other lost souls to Christ; teaching healing classes; ministering in other countries and prison ministry, hospital ministry, and nursing home ministry; ministering to my family members; and doing whatever He has assigned my hands to do. He tells me in II Timothy 1:9, "Who hath saved us, and called us with

an Holy calling, not according to works, but according to His purpose and grace which was given us in Christ Jesus before the world began."
"THAT'S WHY I'VE GOT TO TELL SOMEBODY."

-MY UPPER ROOM EXPERIENCE-

In June of 1984, not quite a year after my first surgery, I received a call from the wife of one of my husband's friends. She invited me to attend a women's retreat that her church was sponsoring for the upcoming weekend. It didn't take much for her to convince me to go when she told me about the Upper Room, where we would be able to go in and pray. However, when she called the church to reserve a seat for me on the bus, they were all taken. Even though I'd never been to this retreat before, I felt an urgency to go like never before. I asked her to call the church again to have them put my name on the waiting list should someone cancel. Within ten minutes, she called me back to inform me that someone had cancelled.

I met her at the church the day of our trip. When I entered the lobby, the members were standing in a circle, singing praise and worship songs and exalting God like I'd never seen before. I loved it so much that I joined the circle, and immediately joy and peace began to fill my heart. I knew at that very moment that I'd never be the same again. This was my first experience with the Pentecostal Church. I'd never seen so many happy people having so much fun serving God. This was also the day I met the pastor, who is a gentle giant for the Lord.

The trip was very exciting, and I knew that this trip was ordained by God. Two other ladies at the hotel joined my friend and I. They, too, were great women of faith. Once we settled in our hotel, we decided that our first visit would be to the Upper Room. As we walked up the pathway to the Upper Room, I noticed the path was covered with stepping stones that had Bible scriptures engraved in each one. As I walked from stone to stone, I began to read their words of wisdom from the Bible, especially Psalms 105, "Thy word is a lamp unto my feet and light unto my path."

Right away, I began to praise God and worship Him in my heart. It was at that moment, I felt that I would never be the same again. "THAT'S WHY I'VE GOT TO TELL SOMEBODY."

-THE PRAYER CLOSET-

When we reached the door of the Upper Room, a lady with the most beautiful smile I'd ever seen opened the door for us to come in. This wasn't my friends' first time coming to the retreat. While the lady was talking to me, each one of them had drifted off to pray or do whatever the Holy Spirit led them to do. I told the lady that I didn't know what to do and that it was my first time there. She asked me if I would like to go into a prayer closet and pray. I said yes. She directed me to sit on the bench in front of the prayer closet doors and wait for someone to come out. Within a few moments, a prayer closet was vacant. I hesitated for a while, remembering that I did not know how to really pray, but the power of God drew me inside. There was an altar with a huge Bible sitting on it, a light shining unusually bright from the ceiling, and a flickering candle-type light on the wall, shining just as bright.

I can remember falling down on my knees in humility, crying out, "Lord, I don't know how to pray. Will you please teach me?"

Now my favorite scripture in the Bible is Psalms 121:1–2 "I will lift up my eyes unto the hills from whence cometh my help, my help cometh from the Lord, who made the Heaven and the Earth." When I looked down at the Bible, it was opened to Psalms 121:1–2. The Spirit of the Lord began to fill my heart and mouth with prayer. I could hear myself praying, but it sounded like someone else. I remember asking God to reveal Himself to me so that I might know that He was truly real.

After I had finished praying, I got up from my knees and attempted to open the door…but the door would not open. Suddenly, the little candle light on the wall began to flicker real fast. I really didn't understand all that was happening, so I just sat down on the bench, which was also the altar, and suddenly, the closet became very warm, and the Spirit of the Lord spoke to my heart saying, "Didn't you ask me to let you feel my presence? Know that I am the Lord."

When I tried again to open the door of the prayer closet, the door opened, and there was the same sweet little lady standing outside the prayer closet again.

She said to me, "Honey, didn't I tell you that you had to go into the prayer closet alone?"

And I said to her, in a troubled voice, "But I was in the prayer closet alone."

Then she looked at me and said, "Okay, honey!"

The moment I came out of the prayer closet, the healing service was beginning. I was so blessed to get a seat on the first bench. I'd never attended a healing service before in my life. Somehow I knew that my blessings were on the way. After a short sermon by the minister, he directed all those who had a serious illness to stand in a line and whisper their sickness into his ear. I was the first in line, so I whispered in his ear that I'd had cancer surgery. He and his assistant anointed my head with oil, and he rebuked that demon of cancer from my body in the name of Jesus. As I walked away, I felt a peace in my heart that I'd never felt before, and I began to cry with joy.

Then a voice said to me, "The cancer and pain in your back from the surgeries will come back."

However, at that point, all the pain in my back and chest was gone, and all I could do was cry and praise God.

-VISITATION OF ANGELS-

I found an empty bench in the back of the upper room that was filled to capacity. The doors were locked so that no one else could go out or come in. As I sat on the bench crying with my back to the service, a woman in a yellow and white striped dress sat down beside me and put her arms around me.

She said, "The Lord told me to tell you not to cry anymore because the cancer is gone."

I said, "But they removed my breast."

"Maybe they didn't have to," she said, and suddenly she was gone.

As the tears streamed down my face, I remembered what the voice had said to me about the pain returning. Suddenly, another woman in a pink- and-white-striped dress kneeled before me and touched me, saying, "If the symptoms return, rebuke them in the name of Jesus." I'd never heard the phase before "I rebuke you in the name of Jesus."

She said, "The Lord told me to tell you to stop crying," and then she was gone without me seeing her face. It was at that point that I realized that I didn't see the first lady's face.

I stopped crying and immediately stood up to look at every woman in the upper room. I was looking for two women, one wearing a yellow-

and-white-striped dress, and another wearing a pink-and-white-striped dress, but I did not see either one of them.

After we left the upper room, I never bothered to tell my roommates about the prayer closet or the women in the upper room, because I was too busy telling them about how the pain in my back and chest was gone. Having told my friends earlier that, because of my physical state, I might not be able to attend all the functions that the church had planned for us, my desire was to go back to the upper room.

I really didn't mind having to stay in the room if the pain got really bad again. Praise God, but He had another plan for my life. I was able to go and enjoy all the functions every day while we were at the retreat.

On the first night, after services, we decided to have Bible study and share something good that God had done for us that day. I shared with them what God had done for me and how the minister had laid hands on me and the pain had left my body. I also told them about my experience in the prayer closet, and the two ladies who came to me with a word from God. Then, through the Spirit of the Lord, one of my roommates began to minister to me regarding the various things that had happened to me in the upper room.

She explained to me that the reason the lady asked me about someone being in the prayer closet with me was because she heard the Lord in my prayer closet, and I felt the warmth of the presence of the Lord in my prayer closet. Furthermore, she explained that the two women who appeared to me were angels.

As for my prayer life, I've been a prayer warrior and a new creation in Christ Jesus every since. Praise the Lord. "THAT'S WHY I'VE GOT TO TELL SOMEBODY."

-A NEW CHILD OF GOD-

After my trip to the retreat, I knew that I'd never be the same. I tried going back to the very quiet church that I'd attended since 1965, but I began to feel that something was missing in my walk with God. It wasn't the fact that I hadn't been baptized, and it wasn't because I did not have a personal relationship with God. It was the fact that I had experienced the touch of Jesus without a doubt.

I realized for the first time in my adult life that He was real in my soul. I realized that He loved me so much that He sent His Heavenly Angels to visit me, to reassure me and confirm my supernatural healing from cancer and back pain so intense that I could hardly bear it sometimes. From that day on, I had no doubt in my heart that I wanted more of Him and I never wanted to live without Him in my life. "THAT'S WHY I'VE GOT TO TELL SOMEBODY."

-STEPPING OUT BY FAITH-

After the retreat, my friend invited me to her church. So with my husband's approval, I attended her church the next Sunday. When I walked through the door of that church, I felt the same presence that was in my prayer closet at the retreat. Without a doubt, I knew this was where God wanted me to be. Within a month, I had become a member of the Church of God, where I received the baptism of the Holy Spirit, joined the choir, and started attending the Bible training classes. But most of all, I was blessed with an awesome relationship with my Heavenly Father. I learned how to bless the Lord at all times with all that is within me...and to bless His holy name.

The day I joined the church, I knew in my spirit that this was God's will. The pastor's message was regarding surrendering to the will of God. About the time, he extended the hand of fellowship for new members. I found myself in the pulpit shaking the pastor's hand.

He said to me, "Welcome Sister Bush."

Since that moment, I've been running, shouting, speaking in tongues, testifying, and praising God in the highest and being a witness for the Lord everywhere I go, winning lost souls for Christ. I am determined to go where He wants me to go, do what He wants me to do, say what He wants me to say, and be who He wants me to be. In my heart, I believe that God is not through with me yet.

On my way home, I realized that I had not talked with my husband about us possibly joining the Church of God. In contemplation of that fact, I remembered my mother always told me that God is not a God of confusion.

So I began to pray, "Oh, Lord, you got me into this, so I'm depending on your grace and mercy to prick my husband's heart so that we can be in agreement with each other."

When I arrived home, my husband was in bed because he was tired from working over the weekend. He had retired from the Air Force and was in his second career on the Capitol Hill Police Force, which he retired from after twenty years of service.

I whispered a prayer and said, "Okay, Father, you said in your word that you are not a God of confusion, so here goes." I tried my best to explain to him what had happened to me.

He just sat up, looked at me, and said, "Honey, if this is where you feel God is leading you, that is wonderful, but I am going to stay at Emmanuel, if that is okay with you."

I just stood there and cried. Once again, God had proven "himself" strong to me. My husband and I attended different churches for about six years. We touched and agreed that God knew what He was doing better than we did.

Although we were attending separate churches, we would visit each other's church often. Mostly it was when I sang solos, led the choir, or participated in large productions during the World Leadership Conferences. During those six years, there was never a moment of confusion. Then one Sunday, the group that God had ordained me to raise, called God's Witness, was singing. My husband was there with our granddaughter, Cristina. When the evangelist finished preaching, he opened the doors of the church to receive new members. Without a warning, my husband grabbed Cristina by the hand and said, "Come on, Chris."

"Where are you going?" I asked.

He looked at me and said, "We are going to join the church."

I said, "I want to go with you."

'Well, you'd better come on," he said.

What a day that was for my husband and I. God had kept His promise when He said he's not a God of confusion. "THAT'S WHY I'VE GOT TO TELL SOMEBODY."

-LEARNING TO LEAN ON THE LORD-

O nce I surrendered my life to the Lord, I began to hunger for His word like never before. One night while sleeping, I had a vision of a scroll going around and around with the 121 Psalms in its entirety. I immediately awakened and could repeat every word verbatim! It was about 1:15 in the morning, and from that night on, for approximately six months, I would awaken at that same time every morning, get up, get my Bible, and go into the kitchen to study.

I used to fumble from one book to another before I could find the book I was looking for. However, now I sat down and boldly read the verses that the Spirit of the Lord reveals to me, with no hesitation at all. It just seemed as though the pages were just being blown open to where the Holy Spirit wanted me to read! Today I thank God's Holy Spirit for anointing me, teaching me, correcting me, cleansing me, healing me, and making me acceptable for my Father in Heaven in Jesus' name.

One of the greatest lessons I learned during that time comes from II Timothy 2:15. "Study to show thyself approved unto God, a workman that need not be ashamed rightly dividing the word of truth." It's so good to know that Psalms 119:105 tells us that "God's word is a lamp unto our feet and a light unto our path."

It was as though the Holy Spirit had set aside those special months to teach the word of God to a sinner like me. I believe with all my heart that this is what He did and that this was God's plan for me before I was conceived in my mother's womb. I call these wonderful blessing "God's Special Plan" and "God's Special Timing" for my life.

Oh how I loved my pastor, a gentle giant for God. He taught me and encouraged me to be all that God would have me be. Soon I began to grow in God's power and might like never before. When I learned how to lift my hands unto the Lord and praise Him, I received the baptism of the Holy Spirit with the evidence of speaking in tongues. I know that He is my gentleness, my fortress, my temperance, my fountain of living waters that never shall run dry, my peace in the midst of a storm, my peace that surpasses all understanding, all that I am, all that I ever shall be, and all that I ever hope to be. He's my all in all. "THAT'S WHY I'VE GOT TO TELL SOMEBODY."

-WALKING IN VICTORY-

A lot of God's people believe that once they have been saved, delivered, healed, Holy-Ghost-filled and fire baptized, their troubles are all over. However, in reality, the Word of God tells us in Ephesians 6:12, "For we wrestle not against flesh and blood but against principalities and powers, against the rulers of darkness of this world and against spiritual wickedness in high places." The moment we choose to serve Jesus is the same moment that the battle has truly just begun.

Satan sends his forces against us with the spirits of disease, afflictions, and infirmities. But don't you fear; God has not given us a spirit of fear, but He has given us a spirit of power, love, and a sound mind. He also promised us that the victory is ours when the battle is His. James 4:7 tells us to "Submit yourselves unto God, resist the devil and he will flee from you." Ephesians 6:12 tells us, "For we wrestle not against flesh and blood, but against principalities, against powers, against the rulers of darkness of spiritual wickedness in high places."

The moment we receive our healing, financial blessing, deliverance, etc., Satan is right there, ready to steal our blessings. But what did Jesus say He came to do? John 10:10 tells us that "Satan cometh not but to steal, kill, and destroy; I am come that they might have life and they might have it more abundantly."

Then the Holy Spirit taught me how to be victorious against Satan, his rulers of darkness, and spiritual wickedness in high places, every day of my life through Christ. He taught me how to put on the whole armor of God in Ephesians 6:14–18. "Stand therefore, having your lions girt about with truth, and having on the breastplate of righteousness; and your feet shod with the preparation of the Gospel of peace, and above all, taking the shield of faith, wherewith ye shall be able to quench all the fiery darts of the wicked. And take the helmet of salvation, and the sword of the Spirit, which is the Word of God; praying always with all prayer and supplication in the Spirit, and watching and waiting thereunto with all perseverance and supplication for all saints." I learned that Satan doesn't come against you when he has you trapped in his camp. But when Jesus sets you free from his hellish camp, that's when the battle begins and he is determined to destroy you. But praise God. It is so good to know that the victory is ours when the battle is the Lord's.

Satan tried to destroy our marriage when we were in two different churches. It wasn't easy sometimes, but God kept us. We had to stay on our knees almost every day, interceding for each other, but God didn't tell us that things were going to be easy. In His own time, God brought us to where He had predestined us to be. My prayer for every man, woman, boy, and girl who reads my life story is that the Spirit of the Lord will anoint you, teach you, correct you, cleanse you, heal you, and make you acceptable for Him in Jesus' name.

I know, without a doubt, that God has graciously opened the windows of Heaven for my husband and I, our children, grandchildren, and great-grandchildren, and our cup overflows. I know, without a doubt, as we stand on Psalms 23:6, "Surely God's goodness and mercy shall follow us all the days of our lives and we shall dwell in the house of the Lord for forever."

I believe, with all my heart that God is just waiting for you to draw nigh to Him so that He can draw nigh to you. I know that if He did it for a sinner like me, then He'll do it for you. "THAT'S WHY I'VE GOT TO TELL SOMEBODY."

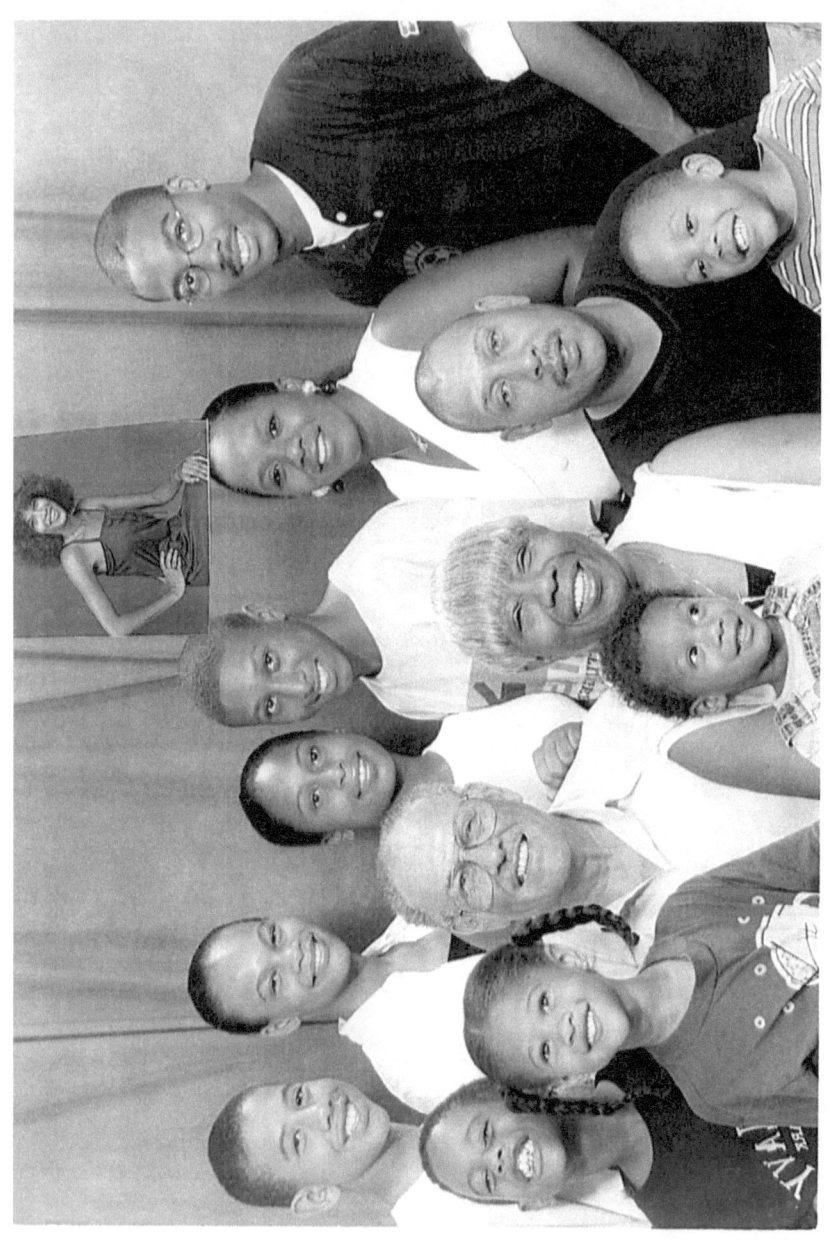

Fannie and Art Bush with Children and Grandchildren

-STANDING ON GOD'S WORD-

After God healed me from cancer in 1983, I was determined in my heart to serve Him all the days of my life. I didn't really understand the Bible as I should have at forty-nine years old, and I had no idea of what walking by faith meant. All I knew was that I was brought up in a Christian home with my mother and stepfather, my precious jewels, who lead me, as best they knew how, in the path of righteousness.

My mom taught us the Bible as best she knew how, constantly reminding us of how much Jesus loved us. When I was young, I totally ignored what she was trying to tell me because it wasn't as exciting or important to me as other worldly things. It wasn't until I came to know Jesus for myself, and He whispered to my heart by way of a disease called cancer and said, "You will not die but live to declare my works." But I want you to remember this:

"Those whom I love, I discipline."

There is a Bible verse that my mother instilled in us and insisted that we learn: John 3:16. "For God so loved the world that he gave His only Begotten Son that whosoever believeth on Him should not perish but shall have everlasting life."

At first, I couldn't understand why God would choose to heal a sinner like me, when for so many years I'd ignored Him and had been disobedient to Him. Then the Holy Spirit quickened me to John 3:16. I know now that if that demon of cancer had killed me in that state I was in spiritually, I would've died in my sins and gone to hell, never to have everlasting life with our Father.

I've since learned that God is merciful, and He is a God of second chances. He looked beyond my faults and saw my needs. The moment I realized what God had done for me, I began to humble myself to Him and repent of my sins. One day, I called my pastor and asked him if I could come over and talk with him. I wanted him to pray with me, touching and agreeing with me, in the name of Jesus, to be saved, delivered, healed, Holy-Ghost-filled and fire-baptized through the blood of Jesus Christ forever. That day, as we prayed, I received deliverance from all of my sins as he interceded for me on my behalf.

I became involved with a special prayer group of godly women on Friday nights, constantly studying to show myself approved unto God. The more I drew nearer to God, the more He drew nearer to me. I learned what it means to walk by faith and not by sight. My most unforgettable miracle of faith was when God delivered me from breast cancer, not once, but twice. During this period of time, I learned that if I desired to keep my healing, than I had to learn how to stand on God's word by faith, and that faith cometh by hearing the word of God all of the time and not some of the time.

Today, I stand on God's Holy Word in II Peter 12:24 and Psalms 118:17–18. I then began to relentlessly seek God's will for my life daily. And today, I constantly stand firmly on Luke 11:9–10, asking, seeking, knocking; and God's constantly opening His door unto me. "THAT'S WHY I'VE GOT TO TELL SOMEBODY."

-ONLY BY GOD'S GRACE-

There have been times in my life when I've asked God to end my suffering, as Paul did in II Corinthians 12:8–10: "Three times I pleaded with the Lord to take this thron away from me, but He said to me, 'My grace is sufficient for you, for my power is made perfect in weakness so that Christ's power may rest on me, For when I am weak, then I am strong."

But then I looked around and I saw people, especially little children, who were suffering much more than I, and all I could do was to look up to Jesus and cry out, "Oh, Lord, thank you for your grace and mercy, which is sufficient for me with the confidence in knowing that your grace is sufficient also for the little children and for all who believe."

I remember my mother always saying to me, "He won't allow you to suffer no more than you can bear, baby."

Then I began to understand Job when he declared in Job 13:15–16, "Though he slay me, yet will I hope in Him. Indeed this will turn out for my deliverance, for no godless man would have come before me."

And it felt so wonderful, like Job, to know that my soul was anchored in the Lord and gripped a solid rock, and that rock is Jesus. He has been truly my lily of the valley, my bright and morning star, my rose of Sharon, the air I breathe, every step I take, every move I make, the fairest of ten thousand to my soul.

When I think about how God has brought me through all the sickness and pain in my life, I stand in awe and amazed by Him. He has been so good to me, and it is all because of God's grace that He has brought me through victories from:

- Crippling Rickets from the age of three to five

- Tonsils removed at the age of six

- Hysterectomy after the birth of our second child

- Back surgery in 1971

- Four breast biopsies

- Back surgery in 1975 twice

- Wrist surgery

- Pain Pump Implant

- Pain Pump Removal

- Toe surgery, four times

- Deviated Septum

- Knee arthroscopic surgery, four times

- Knee cap replacement

- Heart catheterization – three times

- Surgery over entire mouth

- Throat surgery at University of Oklahoma Hospital

- Breast cancer in 1983 and 1985, with no chemo or radiation

- Surgery under right arm because of suspicious growth of cancer; no cancer

- Biopsy of muscle on right arm

- Removal of non-cancerous growth on back

- Surgery of bladder, twice

- Surgery of left rotator cuff from car accident

- Back surgery, upper back, for ruptured vertebrae and crushed vertebrae

- Eye surgery to remove group of small tumors that had accumulated under both eyes over a period of years

- Back surgery for ruptured disk and damaged vertebra pushing against spinal cord

- Bone removed from hip to complete back surgery

- Stomach wrap as a result of Hiatal Hernia, three times

- Torn rotator cuff surgery on both shoulders, 2007

I would get so downhearted whenever I was told that I had to have surgery, not to mention the countless times I've had to have stitches because of accidents. I was a rough tomboy when I was growing up, but God kept me. "THAT'S WHY I'VE GOT TO TELL SOMEBODY."

-WALKING BY FAITH AND NOT BY SIGHT-

One of the most awesome demonstrations of God's healing power (please don't get me wrong because everything that Jesus died for, for us, is awesome) was my back surgery in 2004, which was devastating to me. I had two ruptured vertebrae and one crushed vertebrae in my lower back. After surgery, I began to feel abnormal because of my inability to raise my toes from the ground or twist my ankle in order to walk normally. I was informed that the nerves in my right foot were damaged beyond repair.

As a result of this nerve damage, I developed a condition called Neuropathy, which, according to the doctors, could not be corrected.

"Get on with your life as a cripple, with a condition called (drop foot) the doctor said to me coldly. "There is nothing I can do to help you."

As a result of the doctor's diagnosis, along with the test they ran, I was referred to the physical therapy unit.

The first day I was evaluated by the physical therapist, he informed me that the nerves in my foot were dead. Therefore, I would have to wear a brace on my leg and foot for the rest of my life.

I, in turn, looked at him straight in his eyes and said, "No, I will not."

He looked back at me authoritatively and said, "What makes you think you won't have to wear a brace for the rest of your life?"

I, in turn, looked at him with the name of Jesus as confirmation in my eyes and a "By Jesus stripes I was healed" in my heart, and replied, "Because God didn't make me that way." *Hallelujah!*

This incident occurred in 2004, and today I walk without a brace. I can raise my toes from the ground, and my ankle moves freely. Now, if I had accepted what the physical therapist called down on me and not what was hidden in my heart (God's word), then today I would be walking in defeat. I know, without a doubt, that Jesus took that drop foot on His back once and for all over two thousand years ago. Hallelujah! I will never give Satan the satisfaction of repeating his diagnosis on me again, because by Jesus stripes, I was healed.

Today, I continue to speak the living and healing word of God to my body, my soul, and my spirit every day as I stand steadfast and immovable.

-VISION OF LIFE-

I can remember so well when I had my third stomach wrap, about two and half years ago, in Charlotte, North Carolina. At that moment, I was certain that God was calling me home to be with Him. This was the third surgery for the same problem, a Hiatal hernia in my stomach causing gastric acids to burn the lining of my esophagus, which could eventually cause cancer in my throat. The surgery lasted five hours. I remember being so sick and in so much pain when I awoke two days later. I had tubes in my nose, throat, stomach, neck, and arms. I had been cut from my breast all the way down to the end of my stomach...but God kept.

The first two nights it seemed as though I was fighting for my life. It was during that first night that God gave me a vision. It was as though I was watching a television screen with a bright light. I saw the church bus drive up to our door to drop my husband and I from a church function. When we got inside the house, my husband went into the bedroom to dress for bed, when suddenly, the doorbell ring. When I opened our door, there was a crowd of people standing there. They were all black and featureless! They had no hair, no eyes, no nose, no mouth, no fingers, and no toes. They didn't say anything to me; they just came in and took over our living room, dining room, and kitchen. I could tell who the children were at different ages, who the grownups were, and who the little babies were. They just invaded our home.

62

I cried out to them, "Who are you? What do you want? Why are you doing this to us?"

But they never responded and just continued to disrupt our home.

Then my husband came out of the bedroom and went into our guest bathroom. All of a sudden, one of them went over and stood at the bathroom door, watching him. It was then that I saw the side of its face in the light. It had huge eyes and long eyelashes. When I saw this, I screamed for Art to close the bathroom door.

"Honey, they are looking at you. Close the door. They are watching you!" I screamed.

Then, in the blink of an eye, they were gone! The next day when I saw my husband, I didn't tell him anything because I thought it was just a dream.

The next night, I seemed to be hurting worse and that same light, the one I'd seen the night before, reappeared. I could recognize very well who were the fathers, the mothers, the teenagers, and the little babies. This time the fathers kept throwing the babies up in the air, letting them fall to the floor, but somehow they seemed to land on their feet and hands.

Then I began to cry out, "What do you want? Why are you doing this?" But they would not answer me.

All of a sudden, the screen got larger and brighter. At that point, I looked ahead into the light, and there were two men walking towards the bright light. On my left was a man dressed in a suit, wearing a Stetson hat, with shoes all the same color. It was exactly the way my dad used to dress. The other man, to my right, was dressed in dress pants and a long-sleeved dress shirt. I remember wondering, *who are they?* and my focus was totally on them. Then the Spirit told me to look behind me, and I did. Upon doing so, I saw what seemed to be fire coming up from the earth at the foot of my hospital bed. It seemed to be a burning pit, and the creatures that were in our home were falling into the pit.

I asked the Holy Spirit, "Who are they?"

He said they were the demons that were in our home being cast into the pit of hell from whence they came. He explained that if I had died that first night, or that night, I would have gone straight to hell with the demons.

I seemed to be asking Him the question, "Why?"

-HOLDING UNFORGIVENESS-

The Holy Spirit explained that I was holding unforgiveness in my heart against one of my choir members and that I must go to that person and ask them for forgiveness. He reminded me that unforgiveness cannot enter the Kingdom of Heaven, and then He reminded me that if I had died that first night, I would've opened my eyes in hell.

All of a sudden, I awakened and there was a bright light in the room… but it was the doctors who were leaving my room because I was out of danger. I looked to the right of my bed, and there was my husband standing beside me. He looked as though he had been crying.

I reached up, took his hand, and said, "Honey, I've got to tell you something."

"Go to sleep now, honey; everything is all right," was his response.

Then I began to cry out to him, "But I've got to tell you something, please."

"All right, sweetheart, tell me," he said.

Then, as I began to tell him about the vision, he crawled into the bed, curled up behind me, and listened.

All of a sudden, he said, "Honey, I know what you're talking about."

And that was the last thing I heard him say before I was sound asleep. To this day, I've never asked him what he meant when he said, "Honey, I know what you're talking about." I only know that the Holy Spirit will reveal, through my husband, what he meant when he said, "Honey, I know what you're talking about." Amen.

When I arrived home from the hospital and started going back to church, I called my friend and asked her to forgive me for holding unforgiveness against her in my heart. She told me that she didn't remember making the hurtful statement to me. Oh, what a joy I felt in my heart to know that we were both free. So I witnessed to her about the vision God had given me, and just talking about it in love gave us both that peace that passeth all understanding. That was the day I realized that God had set me free from the spirit of unforgiveness. *"THAT'S WHY I'VE TO TELL SOMEBODY."*

-WORTHY OF THE TEST-

From that time on, I was just being blessed and healing wonderfully. Then one Sunday morning, as I was coming out of church, one of my choir members was waiting for me at the door. He gave me a tape he had purchased at a concert the night before.

"Sister Bush," he said, "I was determined to stand at the door until you came out of church today. Actually, I came early this morning to give you this tape when Brother Bush would let you off at the door as he always does. I wanted to make sure I gave you this tape. But you were already in church, so I thought that I'd wait for you after church."

I didn't respond, so he continued, "The Lord spoke to my heart to give you this tape."

I looked down at the tape and simply said, "Okay."

Then he said, "The third song is yours, Sister Bush!"

Then I graciously took the tape.

When I got in our car, I stuck the tape into the tape deck and switched it over to track three and began to listen to the song. I immediately began to cry, and my husband asked me, "Honey, what's wrong?"

And all I could do was to tell him to listen to the words of the song.

"Your life's been put on hold by some news that you've been given. You've hardly passed the state of unbelief. You've given your life to Jesus but you can't help but thinking, how could He let this happen? How could He let this be? You wonder why God has led you down this path of sorrow, you're worried and oh so afraid. You dread the thought of thinking of what life holds tomorrow, and you hardly have the strength to face the day.

"You've found favor with the Father. He's not angry with you but He needed someone He could trust to let His grace see them through. Don't bow your head in sorrow; don't lay down in regret. You've been chosen for this honor. God has found you worthy of the test.

"Don't believe your life is over. God has not left you behind, so let His armor be what settles the battle raging in your mind - for there's a purpose and a reason for your trials and your test. You can rest assured that God has not finished with you yet."

The next day, I was determined to find out how to get the words of this awesome and anointing song. I wanted to sing it before giving my testimony to the church regarding the vision God had given me.

The first thing I did was look at the soundtrack cover to get a telephone number of the music store that sold the tape. When I found the number to the store, I called to find out whether or not they sold the soundtrack of this particular song. The young lady I talked with was so wonderful.

She informed me that the singing group had the soundtracks but were not ready to sell them yet. Well, at that point, I just broke down and cried as I began to give her my testimony.

Before I could finish, she said to me, "Ms. Fannie, I'll tell you what. I'll give you the name of the young lady who's singing the song, her home number, and her husband's cell phone number in case you can't reach her at home."

Hallelujah!

The same day I called her, we began to share the love of the Lord as though we had known each other for years. After I'd shared my testimony with her, I told her that I would pay her anything she asked for the cost of the track.

"I tell you what, Ms. Fannie," she said, "I'll send you the soundtrack free, and by the way, do you have the book *Jesus the Healer*?"

I said, "No, I don't."

"I'll send that book, too," she said.

Three days later I received a package in the mail from her. About six months later, God blessed my husband and I with the pleasure of attending her concert at another church in our hometown. What a blessing it was.

About two Sundays later, I was scheduled to give my testimony and sing, "Worthy of the Test." This particular morning, I was warming up my voice in our office/music room before my husband and I left for church. In my spirit, I was still puzzled about the two men in the vision. All of a sudden, like before, the vision and bright light reappeared. Once again, I could see the two men going into the bright light. The man I thought was my father was stilled dressed in his same attire, and the man to my right wore the white shirt and dress pants. They were both walking toward the light.

However, this time, the man in the white shirt was rolling down his sleeves as though he had been fighting a battle and was victorious. Like before, I was told to look behind me. When I did, I saw fire coming out of a pit that was at the foot of my hospital bed. The creatures that were in our home were in the pit of fire, but this time I wasn't in the bed.

As I looked toward the two men again, I asked who they were. The Spirit of the Lord said to me, "The man on your left in the suit is my Spirit of Grace, and the man rolling up his sleeves to your right is my Spirit of Mercy."

I believe with all my heart that God had dispatched his warring angels to defeat the demons that were in our home. I also believe that because of his Grace and Mercy, it was not His will that I should perish.

-MESSAGE FOR THE CHURCH-

The Spirit of God reminds me every day that this message is not for me to keep to myself. It is for the world because there are so many of God's children who have been walking around with unforgiveness, hate, anger, malice, jealousy, spite, and more for years without realizing that these issues are still buried deep down in their hearts. So many have never gotten down on their knees and asked God to search their hearts every day of their lives, as David did in Psalms 139:23–24, "Search me, Oh God, and know my heart; test me and know my anxious thoughts. See if there is any way in me, and lead me in the way everlasting"; Psalms 51:10, "Create in me a clean heart, O God; and renew a right spirit in me"; and Psalms 51:12, "Restore unto me the joy of my salvation and uphold me with thy free Spirit."

We need to ask God to take away our hearts of stone and give us broken and contrite hearts to serve Him in spirit and in truth all the days of our lives. We need hearts filled with love for each other, just as Christ loves us. He loves us so much that He suffered and died on the Cross of Calvary to pay for our sins - He who was without sin. I beg of you today, in the name of Jesus, to always remember that John 3:16–17 tells it all: "For God so loved the world that He gave His only begotten Son that whosoever believeth on Him should not perish but shall have everlasting life. 'For God sent not His Son into the world to condemn the world, but that the world through Him might be saved." I beg of you today, in the name of Jesus, please don't let His death on the cross be in vain.

The Spirit of the Lord also quickened my heart to the truth that when this vision is revealed to every saint and sinner, there will not be enough room at the altar for those who will be coming to surrender their lives to Jesus. What a day that will be when all of those whose hearts are being convicted by the Holy Spirit are set free at last. What a day that will be when that old spirit of eating cancer will once and for all be thrown into the pit of hell forever. And because, God is no respecter of persons, we can all pray as David did and ask for a clean heart, a broken and contrite heart, to serve Him for the rest of our days. Hallelujah!

I pray every day for you that you refuse to allow the spirit of pride to stop you from surrendering your body, soul, and spirit totally and completely to the Father. He is not going to force you, but He surely will receive you unto Himself when you surrender your all to Him.

I don't know about you, but Jesus said that He is coming back again for a church without a spot or wrinkle, and, according to Ephesians 5:27, "To present to Him a church, without a spot or wrinkle *or any other blemish*."

I want to be ready when Jesus comes for His Bride, should I be alive— but if not, you can rest assured that I'll be somewhere around His Throne with Him in Heaven. I'll be among that great cloud of witnesses just rooting for you on this earth. "THAT'S WHY I'VE GOT TO TELL SOMEBODY."

-MY SOUL'S DESIRE-

Revelation 12: 11 tells us "And they overcame Him by the Blood of the Lamb, and by the words of their testimony." For this reason, I believe that God has allowed me to live, move, breathe, and have my being, to be saved, delivered, healed, Holy-Ghost-filled, and fire-baptized, and to be known by the blood of the Lamb and the word of my testimony.

How do you know all of this, Sister Bush? Well, God's word tells me, according to Romans 8:9, "For whom He did foreknow, He also did predestine to be conformed to the image of His Son." And according to Romans 8:30, "More over whom He also did predestinate them also He justified."

Today, my soul's desire is to continue to do God's will and be the witness that God would have me be in this world. You see, it is no longer I who lives but it is Christ who lives in me. I know with all my heart that it is God's perfect will that I write this precious book so that this message can reach the unreachable—those who would never be saved, delivered, healed, Holy-Ghost-filled, and fire-baptized had I not been obedient to Him.

The Lord has quickened me to the fact that many of His people in this world, who He has healed, are still hiding their lights under bushes. They are hiding as a result of their fear of rejection, ashamed of the

Gospel because of lack of knowledge, no holy boldness, and a lack of the knowledge of knowing that God has not given them a spirit of fear. But He has given them a spirit of power and love, and a sound mind, as well as life abundantly and a testimony. I challenge you today to study God's word and hear the heartbeat of God, our Father, and stand on His holy word in John 14:12–13, "Verily, verily I say unto you, He that believeth on me, the works that I do shall he do also and greater works shall he do because I go unto the Father and whatsoever ye ask in my name, that will I do, that the Father may be glorified in the Son."

Don't continue to allow Satan to steal your testimony about what God had done for you—*TELL SOMEBODY.* Write a book. Pray and let God's Holy Spirit increase the gifts in you for God to receive the glory. Then you too will live, and not die, to declare the works of the Lord. Stay in God's word. Please don't be ashamed to confess to the world every day how you were healed by Jesus' stripes. And be very bold in your confession and testimony.

Don't allow the devil to stop you from witnessing to others about what God has done for you. THAT'S WHY I'VE GOT TO TELL SOMEBODY'

If He's healed you supernaturally,

'YOU'VE GOT TO TELL SOMEBODY."

If He's healed you in the natural,

"YOU'VE GOT TO TELL SOMEBODY"

If He's saved your soul and made you whole again,

"YOU'VE GOT TO TELL SOMEBODY"

But, most of all, if you know that you're on your way to heaven,

"YOU'VE GOT TO TELL SOMEBODY"

Without Him in the midst of it all, none of these miracles would be possible. Jesus reminded His disciples in Mark 9: 39–41, "No man that does a miracle in my name can, in the next moment, say anything bad about me, for whoever is not against us is for us."

So I ask you a question, If God has saved your soul, healed you, and made you whole again, delivered you from evil, and you're living, moving, breathing and having your being, are you for Him or against Him?

If your answer is, "Yes" you're for Him, then get out and, "TELL SOMEBODY."

MAY THE LORD BLESS YOU AND KEEP YOU - MAY HE CAUSE HIS FACE TO SHINE UPON YOU AND GIVE YOU LOVE, JOY, PEACE, HEALING AND HOLY BOLDNESS NOW HENCEFORTH AND FOREVERMORE IN JESUS' PRECIOUS, HOLY, AND RIGHTEOUS NAME.

AMEN AMEN & AMEN